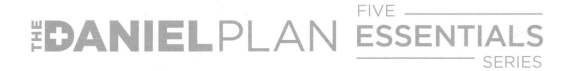

THE **DANIEL** PLAN · FIVE ESSENTIALS SERIES

FOCUS

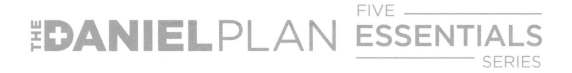

THE DANIEL PLAN

FIVE
ESSENTIALS
SERIES

FOCUS

Essential Four

RENEWING YOUR MIND

STUDY GUIDE   FOUR SESSIONS

featuring

DR. DANIEL AMEN
& DEE EASTMAN

with KAREN LEE-THORP

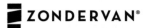

ZONDERVAN®

ZONDERVAN

Focus Study Guide
Copyright © 2015 by The Daniel Plan

This title is also available as a Zondervan ebook. Visit www.zondervan.com/ebooks.

Requests for information should be addressed to:
Zondervan, 3900 *Sparks Dr. SE, Grand Rapids, Michigan 49546*

ISBN 978-0-310-88958-8

All Scripture quotations, unless otherwise indicated, are taken from The Holy Bible, *New International Version®, NIV®.* Copyright © 1973, 1978, 1984, 2011 by Biblica, Inc.® Used by permission. All rights reserved worldwide.

Scripture quotations marked NLT are taken from the *Holy Bible, New Living Translation,* copyright © 1996, 2004. Used by permission of Tyndale House Publishers, Inc., Wheaton, Illinois. All rights reserved.

Scripture quotations marked MSG are taken from *The Message.* Copyright © 1993, 1994, 1995, 1996, 2000, 2001, 2002. Used by permission of NavPress Publishing Group.

Any Internet addresses (websites, blogs, etc.) and telephone numbers in this book are offered as a resource. They are not intended in any way to be or imply an endorsement by Zondervan, nor does Zondervan vouch for the content of these sites and numbers for the life of this book.

Cover photography: iStockphoto
Interior photography: Robert Ortiz, Kent Cameron, Don Haynes, Robert Hawkins, Shelly Antol, Matt Armendariz,
    the PICS Ministry at Saddleback Church, iStockphoto
Interior design: Kait Lamphere

First Printing May 2015 / Printed in the United States of America

Contents

Welcome Letter   6

How to Use This Guide   7

SESSION 1
Brain Health   11

SESSION 2
Mindset Matters   27

SESSION 3
Breaking through Barriers   43

SESSION 4
Don't Mess with Stress   61

APPENDIX

Biblical Meditation   81

Identifying ANTs   85

Keeping Sabbath   87

Group Guidelines   89

Leadership 101   91

Memory Verses   95

About the Contributors   97

Welcome Letter

I am so glad you have joined us for this Daniel Plan study. I am excited for your journey, as I have seen firsthand that change is within reach as you embrace the Daniel Plan lifestyle. This groundbreaking program will equip you with practical tools to bring health into every area of your life. It has been transformative for thousands of people around the world and can be for you as well.

I speak from experience. I've not only witnessed endless stories of life change but have personally benefited from these Daniel Plan Essentials for many years now. Working full-time with five grown children, including identical triplet girls, I understand what it is like to juggle many priorities and have my health impacted. The key elements of The Daniel Plan have been completely restorative in my life as I have integrated them one step at a time.

As you go through this four-week study, the perfect complement to maximize your success is reading *The Daniel Plan: 40 Days to a Healthier Life*. The book includes a 40-day food and fitness guide, complete with a meal plan, recipes, shopping lists, and exercises that will energize your efforts. It will complement any of The Daniel Plan studies you dive into. There are also numerous articles and free resources on our website (www.danielplan.com), along with a weekly newsletter filled with tools and inspiration to keep you flourishing.

Congratulations on taking the next step to gaining vitality in your life. My prayer is that you will be inspired and fully equipped to continue your journey, and that you will experience a whole new level of wellness in the process. I pray that you will feel God's presence and will be reenergized to follow all he has planned for you.

For His Glory,

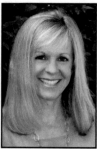

Dee Eastman

Dee Eastman
Founding Director, The Daniel Plan

How to Use This Guide

There are five video studies in The Daniel Plan series, one for each of the five Essentials (Faith, Food, Fitness, Focus, and Friends). Each study is four sessions long. The studies may be done in any order. If your group is new, consider starting with the six-week *The Daniel Plan Study Guide* and companion DVD, which offers an overview of all five Essentials.

GROUP SIZE

Each Daniel Plan video study is designed to be experienced in a group setting such as a Bible study, Sunday school class, or any small group gathering. To ensure that everyone has enough time to participate in discussions, it is recommended that large groups break into smaller groups of four to six people each.

MATERIALS NEEDED

Each participant should have his or her own study guide, which includes notes for video segments, directions for activities, discussion questions, and ideas for personal application between sessions. This curriculum is best used in conjunction with *The Daniel Plan: 40 Days to a Healthier Life*, which includes a complete 40-day food and fitness guide that complements this study.

TIMING

Each session is designed to be completed in 60 to 90 minutes, depending on your setting and the size of your group. Each video is approximately 20 minutes long.

OUTLINE OF EACH SESSION

Each group session will include the following:

» *Coming Together.* The foundation for spiritual growth is an intimate connection with God and his family. A few people who really know you and earn your trust provide a place to experience the life Jesus invites you to live. This opening portion of your meeting is an opportunity to transition from your busy life into your group time.

   In Session 1 you'll find some icebreaker questions on the session topic, along with guidelines that state the values your group will live by so that everyone feels comfortable sharing. In Sessions 2 - 4 you'll have a chance to check in with other group members to report praise and progress toward your goals of healthy living. You'll also be able to share how you chose to put the previous session's insights into practice – and what the results were. There's no pressure for everyone to answer. This is time to get to know each other better and cheer each other on.

» *Learning Together.* This is the time when you will view the video teaching segment. This study guide provides notes on the key points of the video teaching along with space for you to write additional thoughts and questions.

» *Growing Together.* Here is where you will discuss the teaching you watched. The focus will be on how the teaching intersects with your real life.

» *What I Want to Remember.* You'll have a couple of minutes after your discussion to write down one or two key insights from the teaching and discussion that you want to remember.

» *Better Together.* The Daniel Plan is all about transforming the way you actually live. So before you close your meeting in prayer, you'll take some time to think about how you might apply what you've discussed. Under "Next Steps" you'll find a list of things you can do to put the session's insights into practice. Then the "Food Tip of the Week" offers a bonus video with a great recipe or food idea. It is on your DVD if you want to view it together with your group. It is also available online for you to view on your own during the week. Likewise, the "Fitness Move of the Week" is a bonus video with a simple exercise you can add to your fitness practices. It, too, is on your DVD and online.

Encourage each other to be specific about one or two things you plan to do each week as next steps. Consider asking someone in the group to be your buddy to hold each other accountable. Create an atmosphere of fun and positive reinforcement.

» *Praying Together.* The group session will close with time for a response to God in prayer, thanking him for what he's doing for you and asking for his help to live out what you have learned. Ideas for group prayer, as well as a written closing prayer, are provided. Feel free to use them or not. Consider having different group members lead the prayer time.

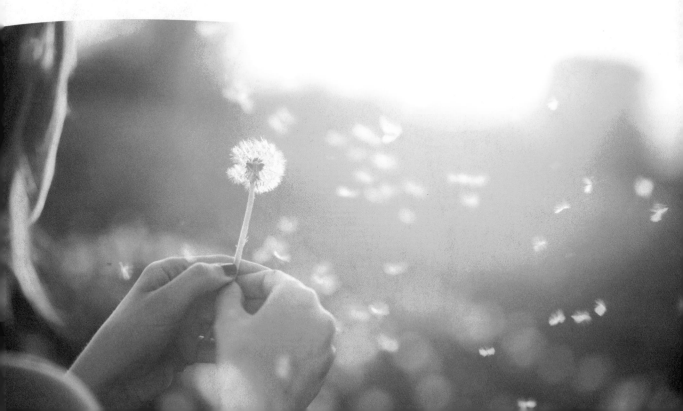

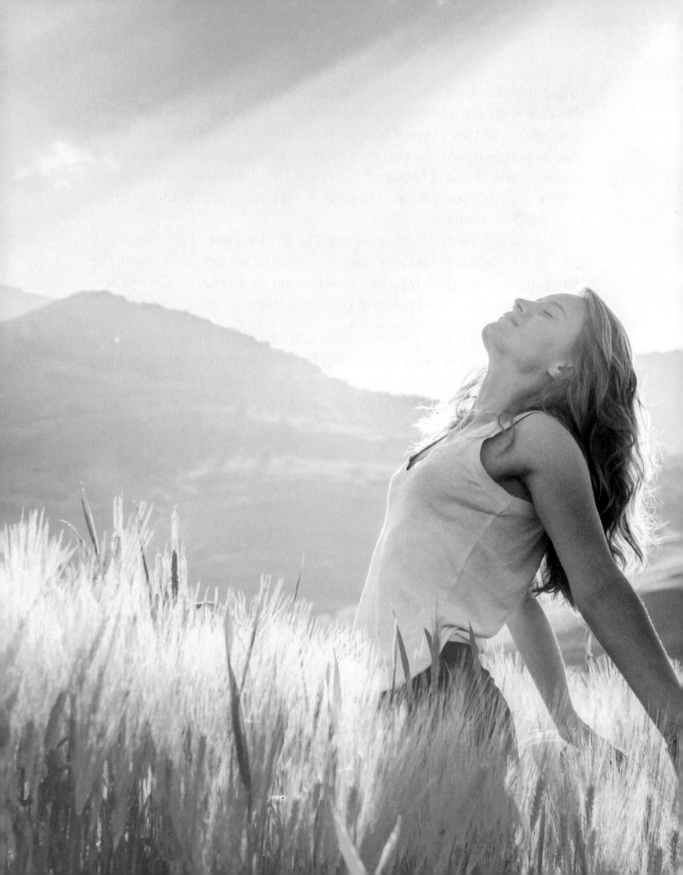

Brain Health

> "My counsel is this: Live freely, animated and motivated by God's Spirit. Then you won't feed the compulsions of selfishness."
> Galatians 5:16 (MSG)

Did you know that our brains are a key component of a healthy lifestyle? Changing the way we eat and exercise requires changing the way we think about food, our bodies, and ourselves. Thinking is a function of our brains, and changing the way we think is easier when we know a few things about how our brains work. In this study on Focus, we'll learn how to get our thoughts right and discover what a transformative effect that can have on our health—in fact, on our whole life.

In addition, just as good thoughts profoundly affect our ability to eat right and get proper exercise, so also having a healthy brain is one of the main reasons to eat healthy food and get exercise. As we'll see in this first session, what we eat affects our risk of brain ailments such as Alzheimer's and even affects the clarity of our day-to-day decision making. Food is medicine for our bodies, and that's especially true for our brains. Brain health and body health—they go hand in hand.

COMING
TOGETHER

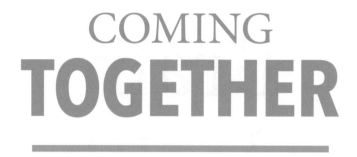

If this is your first time meeting together as a group, take a moment to introduce yourself.

Also, pass around a sheet of paper on which each person can write his or her name, address, phone number, and email address. Ask for a volunteer to type up the list and email it to everyone else this week.

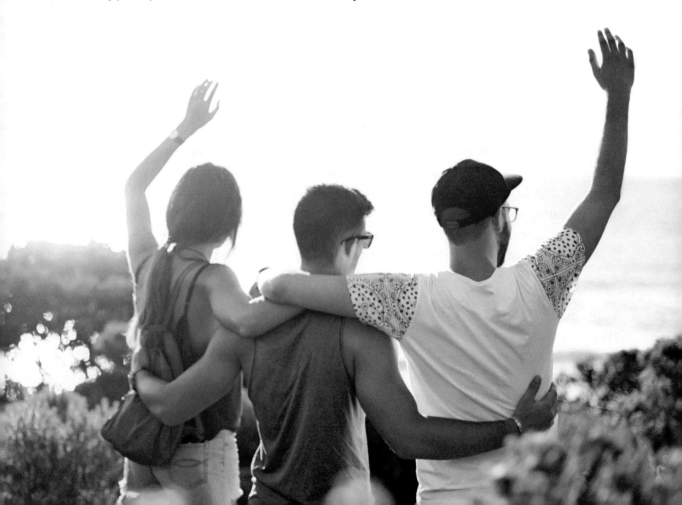

Finally, you'll need some simple group guidelines that outline values and expectations. See the sample in the Appendix and make sure that everyone agrees with and understands those expectations.

When you're finished with these introductory activities, give everyone a chance to respond to this icebreaker question:

» What you think matters to what you do and what results you experience. Share one thing you have been thinking about The Daniel Plan. It can be something positive, such as a good experience or a hopeful or encouraging belief. Or it can be a concern, a question, or a frustration. Just put it out there, whatever is on your mind.

LEARNING
TOGETHER

AN INTERVIEW WITH Dr. Daniel Amen

Play the video segment for Session 1. As you watch, use the outline provided to follow along or to take additional notes on anything that stands out to you.

» Focus is about brain health and getting our thoughts right.

» Our brain is the organ of judgment, personality, character, and every decision that we make. When our brain works right, we work right.

» When our brain is troubled because of a head injury, improper eating, or any other reason, we have trouble in life. We are sadder, sicker, poorer. And we have trouble sticking with a healthy program.

» We need to:

  • Care about our brain

  • Stop doing things that hurt our brain

  • Do things that help our brain

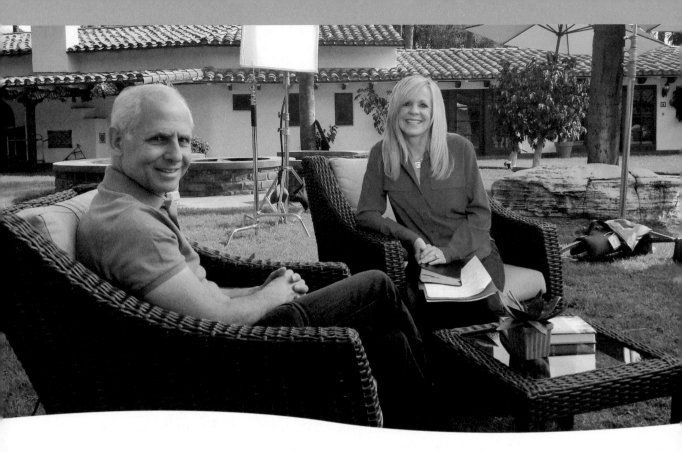

» Things we should stop:

  • Drugs and alcohol

  • Brain injuries in contact sports

  • Obesity (as our weight goes up, our brain size and function go down)

  • High blood sugar (as blood sugar goes up, brain function goes down)

  • High blood pressure

  • Untreated sleep apnea

  • Untreated depression

- Untreated ADD

- Negative thinking (if we think in negative terms, the part of our brain that makes decisions doesn't work as well)

- Inflammation from foods like corn, soy, and sugar

» The brain is only 2 percent of the body's weight, but it uses 20 to 30 percent of the calories we consume and 25 percent of the blood flow. To have good blood flow, we need healthy blood vessels. High blood sugar is associated with blood vessels becoming brittle and breaking.

» Good things for the brain include:

- Aerobic exercise (it increases blood flow)

- Coordination exercises (activities that take coordination—such as dance, table tennis, and juggling—connect new pathways in the brain)

- High-quality protein

- High-quality fat

- Vegetables

- Multi-vitamins

- Vitamin D

- Fish oil

- Gratitude

- Spending time with healthy people

» Where we put our attention determines how we feel. We need to feed our brains with life-giving thoughts, including the truths of Scripture.

» If we write down three things we are grateful for every day, it increases our sense of happiness.

» When we give away good information about healthy living, we create our own support system and make it more likely we will stay on the program. Get it, learn it, and give it away.

» There is no cure for Alzheimer's because it starts in a person's brain thirty to fifty years before they have symptoms. We prevent Alzheimer's by preventing the illnesses associated with it: obesity, heart disease, hypertension, diabetes, depression, sleep apnea.

» You are not stuck with the brain you have. You can make it better.

» Fifty-one percent of Americans will have a challenge with a psychiatric disorder sometime in their lives. Struggling with anxiety, depression, or another disorder is normal. Normal people have problems. The smart ones get help for their problems.

GROWING
TOGETHER

Discuss what you learned from the video. Don't feel obliged to answer every question. Select those that most resonate with your group.

 Why should we care about brain health?

 Look at the list of things we should stop doing in the video notes. Which of those do you need to attend to? How might you go about that?

 "Where we put our attention determines how we feel." How have you experienced this to be true? Think about where you've put your attention during the past day and how your mood has been affected.

"I pray that from his glorious, unlimited resources he will empower you with inner strength through his Spirit."
Ephesians 3:16 (NLT)

Take a moment right now to write down three things you are grateful for.

> *"Enter his gates with thanksgiving and his courts with praise; give thanks to him and praise his name."*
>
> Psalm 100:4

 What can you do to fill your attention with the truths of Scripture? (See the article "Biblical Meditation" in the Appendix.)

 Half of all Americans will struggle with a psychiatric disorder such as depression or anxiety at some time in their lives. How is it helpful for you to know that it's normal to have these struggles? What do you think is an appropriate way to respond to someone we know who has one of these disorders? What do you think we should do if we ourselves struggle with one of these disorders?

> *"For God has not given us a spirit of fear and timidity, but of power, love, and self-discipline."*
>
> 2 Timothy 1:7 (NLT)

 Why is it important to know that we are not stuck with the brains we have? How does it affect you personally to know that?

What I Want
to Remember

Complete this activity on your own.

» Briefly review the video outline and any notes you took. Review also any notes from the discussion.

» In the space below, write down the most significant thing you gained from this session—from the video or the discussion. You can share it with the group if you wish.

BETTER
TOGETHER

Now that you've talked about some great ideas, let's get practical — and put what you're learning into action. The Daniel Plan centers around five essential areas of health. In this study you're exploring Focus, so you can begin by identifying one or two steps you can take for a healthier brain. Then check out the Food Tip of the Week and the Fitness Move of the Week for some fresh ideas to enrich your journey toward health in those areas. There are also many tips and tools on the danielplan.com website so you can keep growing in all of the Essentials while doing this study. Use or adapt whatever is helpful to you!

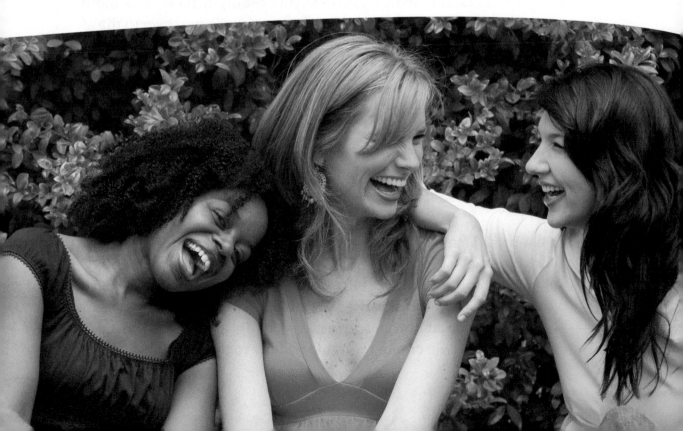

FOCUS
Next Steps

"And let us consider how we may spur one another on toward love and good deeds."
Hebrews 10:24

Here are a few suggested activities to help you pursue brain health. Check one or two boxes next to the options you'd like to try—choose what works for you.

☐ Notice where your attention goes this week. Set a timer on your phone to go off every hour and write down what you were thinking about just before the timer went off. At the end of the week, look for patterns. What do you tend to think about? Do your thoughts tend to be more negative or more positive? How much attention do you give to the things of God or the words of Scripture? Do your thoughts encourage you to love your neighbor? Don't be critical of yourself because of the things you think about. Just take this time to notice, to become aware.

☐ Take time each day this week to fill your attention with a truth from Scripture. See the article "Biblical Meditation" in the Appendix for ideas. See also the Memory Verses in the Appendix. See if you can commit one verse to memory.

☐ Take a break in a busy day to try a breathing exercise to relax your mind. Breathe in for four slow counts, hold for two counts, breathe out for four counts, hold for two counts. Do this ten times. Try to breathe as deeply and slowly as possible. Fill your belly with breath. You'll be amazed at how much calmer you feel afterward. This slow, deep breathing will create more blood flow to the front of your brain.

- [ ] Commit to eating according to The Daniel Plan as a way of pursuing brain health. What is one step you can take, such as eliminating sugar from your diet this week, or eating only healthy fats?

- [ ] Do you snore when you sleep? Make an appointment to talk with your doctor about sleep apnea, a condition in which a person briefly stops breathing during sleep. Sleep apnea reduces blood flow to the brain, so if you have that condition, be aware that it can be treated.

- [ ] Get thirty minutes of aerobic exercise three times this week. It will increase blood flow to your brain.

- [ ] Try a form of exercise that requires coordination, such as dancing, table tennis, or juggling.

- [ ] Ask your doctor to do a blood test for vitamin D. If you haven't had your cholesterol and blood sugar tested recently, do those also.

- [ ] Start taking fish oil, which is full of omega-3 fats that are good for your brain.

- [ ] Write down three things you are grateful for every day this week. Notice how it affects your mood.

Food Tip
of the Week

Eating right is essential to thinking right, and thinking right is essential to living the life God intends for us. This week's food tip focuses on high-quality food for our brains. Try this recipe for a healthy brain smoothie to get your day started well. Just click the Food Tip of the Week on your video screen (3 minutes), scan the QR code, or go to danielplan.com/foodtip.

Fitness Move
of the Week

Do you have discomfort or pain in your lower back? Learn a move to strengthen your back. Just click the Fitness Move of the Week on your video screen (1 minute), use the QR code, or go to danielplan.com/fitnessmove.

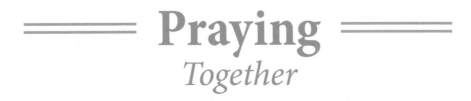

Praying
Together

Because everything we do in our journey toward health depends on God's power, we end each meeting with prayer and encourage group members to pray for each other during the week.

> *"Rejoice always, pray continually, give thanks in all circumstances; for this is God's will for you in Christ Jesus."*
> 1 Thessalonians 5:16–18

This week, offer prayers of gratitude to God. Thank him for the things you wrote down in question 4. Thank him for your brain and what you are learning about it. Give everyone in the group a chance to pray one- or two-sentence prayers of gratitude.

Have someone close with this prayer:

Thank you, Lord, for our brains. Thank you for the intricate ways they work, with a hundred billion nerve cells sending messages all over our bodies. Thank you for giving each of us the capacity to think wisely and make good decisions. Please fill us with your Holy Spirit so that we will have deeper wisdom, and guide us to good decisions to care for our brains. We know that we are profoundly influenced simply by what we think about, so we want to fill our minds with thoughts of you. You are all-powerful, completely loving, and wise in all things. You sent your Son to die for us and rise from the dead. Please fill us anew with the wonder of such thoughts. Thank you for each person in this group. I pray this in Jesus' name. Amen.

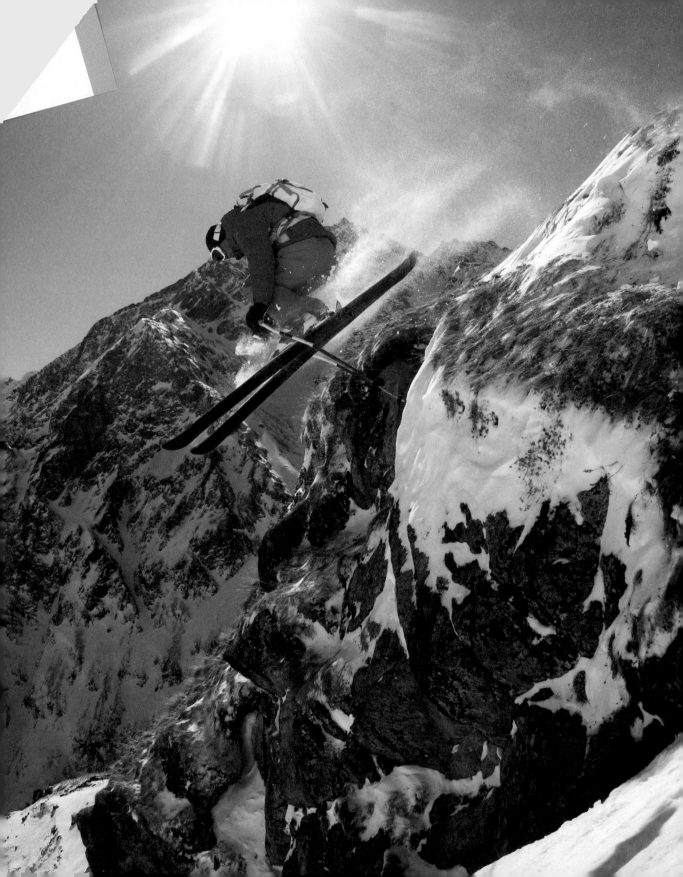

Mindset Matters

> "Finally, brothers and sisters, whatever is true, whatever is noble, whatever is right, whatever is pure, whatever is lovely, whatever is admirable – if anything is excellent or praiseworthy – think about such things."
>
> Philippians 4:8

Do you ever find yourself stuck in negative thinking about something – maybe your body, your fitness, your eating habits, your job, or your marriage? It's so easy to get caught up in negative thoughts that make us feel like we're walking around with ten-pound weights chained to our arms and legs. In this session we'll learn why it's important to unchain those weights and also how we can do it. There are some simple things we can do to change the way we think, and God is eager to help.

COMING
TOGETHER

The other members of your group can be a huge source of support in sustaining healthy changes in your life. Before watching the video, check in with each other about your experiences since the last session. For example:

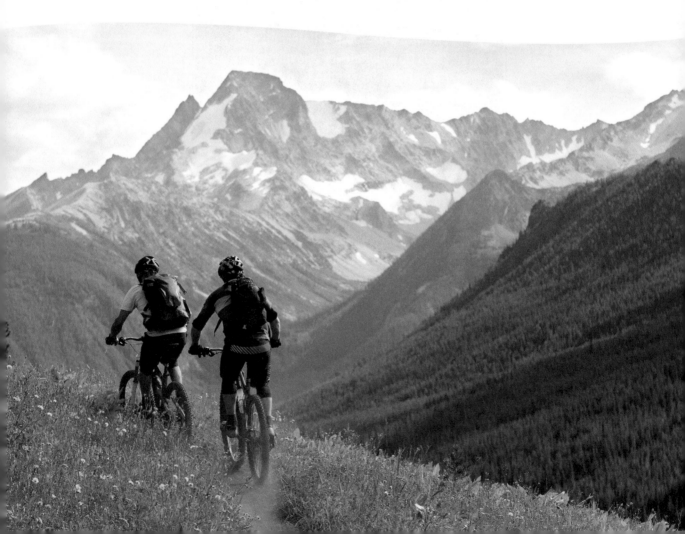

» Briefly share what Next Steps from Session 1 you completed or tried to complete. Were they helpful? If so, how?

» How did Session 1 affect the way you think about and treat your brain?

» Have you been practicing The Daniel Plan in other areas, such as Food or Fitness? If so, what have you done? What is working well for you? What questions do you have? What encouragement do you need?

LEARNING
TOGETHER

AN INTERVIEW WITH Dr. Daniel Amen

Play the video segment for Session 2. As you watch, use the outline provided to follow along or to take additional notes on anything that stands out to you.

"Do not conform to the pattern of this world, but be transformed by the renewing of your mind."
Romans 12:2

» Every time we have a thought, our brains release chemicals. When we have a sad, angry, anxious, hopeless, or helpless thought, our brains release chemicals that make us feel awful. Negative thoughts make our hands colder, our muscles more tense, our breathing shallower, and our brainwaves disorganized.

» When we have a happy, hopeful, encouraging, loving, or connected thought, our brains release a completely different set of chemicals. Our hands get warmer and drier, our muscles become more relaxed, and our breathing becomes slower and deeper.

» Thoughts matter, but they are automatic. We often don't plan them. Yet if we don't correct them, thoughts lie. Our uninvestigated thoughts often steal our happiness and ruin our health.

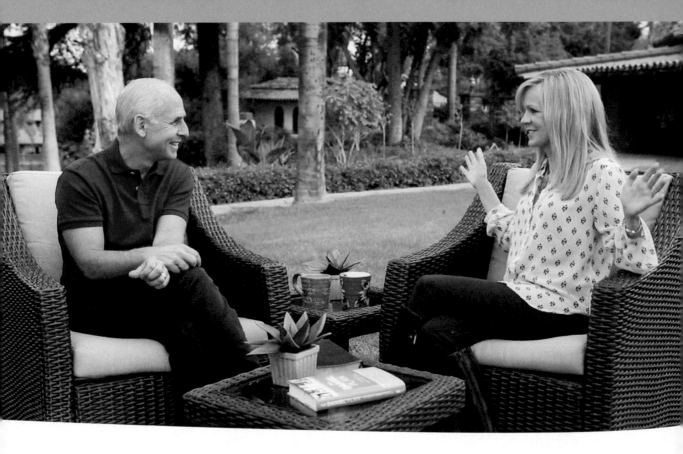

» ANTs stands for *automatic negative thoughts*. These are thoughts that come into our minds automatically and ruin our day. We need to kill the ANTs. We need an internal anteater to patrol the streets of our minds.

» When we reflect on our thoughts and are able to see things more clearly, then we can grow and move forward.

» Learning not to believe every negative thing we think has been shown in research studies to be as effective as antidepressant medication. It has also been shown to be helpful for weight loss, panic attacks, and relationships.

» The exercise for challenging negative thoughts is simple. Whenever you feel sad, mad, nervous, or out of control, write down what you think. Then question your thoughts. Is it true? Just those three words, "Is it true?" can cause a revolution in your life. "The truth will set you free" (John 8:32).

» Then, replace the negative thought with the truth from God's Word. "I had a bad day, but what is true that God says about me? He says I am loved, I am cared for, his strength is made perfect in my weakness. I can approach the throne of grace in confidence and find help in my time of need." (See the article "Biblical Meditation" in the Appendix for a list of Scripture passages that you can meditate on to replace lies with truth.)

» From thousands of stories of transformation, we know that virtually anyone can stay on The Daniel Plan if they get the right mindset. It's not hard. It's not about deprivation. It's not expensive. Being sick is expensive.

» When you do the right thing, stop telling yourself that you are depriving yourself. That false message about deprivation is what gets people off The Daniel Plan. Healthy food is great food. Bad food deprives us of what we really want, which is health.

» If you write down three things you are grateful for every day, within three weeks you will notice a significant increase in your level of happiness.

» Even more powerful is telling three people a day that you appreciate them, and why. By doing that, you feel gratitude for someone and then you give it away.

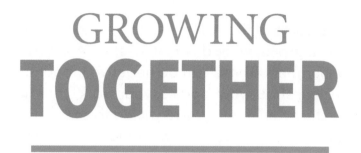

GROWING
TOGETHER

Discuss what you learned from the video. Don't feel obliged to answer every question. Select those that most resonate with your group.

 1 What does Proverbs 4:23 say about our innermost thoughts? Why does it matter if we have chronically negative thoughts?

> *"Above all else, guard your heart,*
> *for everything you do flows from it."*
> Proverbs 4:23

 2 Why do you think Dr. Amen recommends questioning negative thoughts, asking "Is it true?" Why not just suppress the negative thought and make up a positive thought?

3 What are some of the ANTs that come into your head automatically? As a group, write down at least six ANTs from various group members. These can be negative thoughts about The Daniel Plan, about your bodies, your work, your health, your relationships — anything you're willing to share. (For example, "The Daniel Plan is depriving me of food that tastes good.")

4 Question each of the ANTs you wrote down. Ask, "Is it true?" Try to state what is true in each case. Write down the truth regarding each of your own ANTs.

"For we do not have a high priest who is unable to empathize with our weaknesses, but we have one who has been tempted in every way, just as we are — yet he did not sin. Let us then approach God's throne of grace with confidence, so that we may receive mercy and find grace to help us in our time of need."

Hebrews 4:15–16

*"My grace is sufficient for you, for my power
is made perfect in weakness."*
2 Corinthians 12:9

 Review the list of Scripture passages in the article "Biblical Meditation" as well as the Memory Verses in the Appendix. Which passage would be helpful for you to meditate on in order to replace false ANTs with truth? If none of these passages seems ideal, can you think of another passage that is relevant?

 What do you think we should do with negative thoughts that *are* true? What if we are sad about a real loss, for example?

 As Proverbs 17:22 says, "A cheerful heart is good medicine." Take a moment to write down three things you are grateful for— that are good medicine for you.

What I Want
to Remember

Complete this activity on your own.

» Briefly review the video outline and any notes you took. Review also any notes from the discussion.

» In the space below, write down the most significant thing you gained from this session — from the video or the discussion. You can share it with the group if you wish.

BETTER
TOGETHER

Now that you've talked about some great ideas, let's get practical — and put what you're learning into action. Begin by identifying one or two steps you can take in this session on Focus. Then check out the Food Tip of the Week and the Fitness Move of the Week for some fresh ideas to enrich your journey toward health in those areas. Use or adapt whatever is helpful to you!

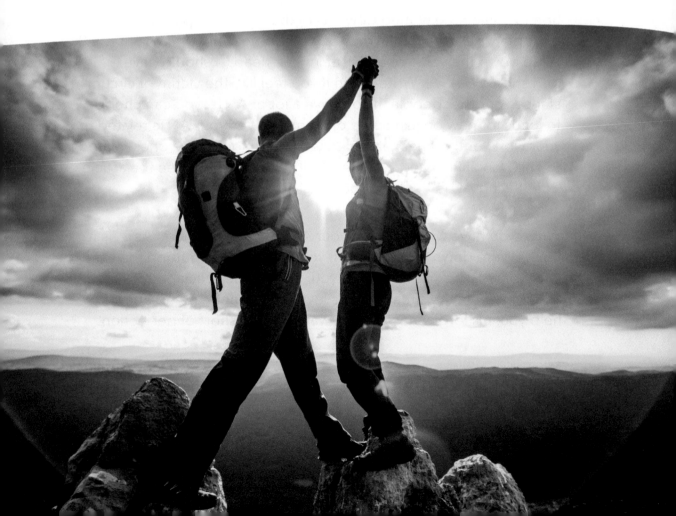

FOCUS
Next Steps

Here are a few suggested activities to help you move forward in shaping a mindset that is grounded in truth. Check one or two boxes next to the options you'd like to try this week—choose what works for you.

☐ Write down three things you are grateful for every day this week.

☐ Tell three people each day that you appreciate them, and why.

☐ Spend some time writing down all of the ANTs that plague you. For example, write down the voice of worry in your head ("What if . . . ?"). Write down the voice of criticism in your head ("I should have . . ." or "I should be . . ."). Write down if you feel like the victim of circumstances or other people. If you have a lot of ANTs, you can choose to focus for now on just some of them, such as your ANTs related to your work, or the ones related to your marriage, or the ones related to The Daniel Plan and your health. If you need help, see the article "Identifying ANTs" in the Appendix.

☐ When you have written down your ANTs, question them. Ask, "Is it true?" Write down what is true. If you have trouble putting the truth into words, ask a friend to help you. Think especially about God's involvement in the situation—his love, his willingness and ability to help you, his forgiveness for the ways you fall short of perfection.

☐ Memorize a Scripture passage that speaks truth that you need to hear. See "Biblical Meditation" and "Memory Verses" in the Appendix. Post your verse somewhere you will see it multiple times a day. Read it aloud until you have committed it to memory.

☐ Get together with a friend to help each other replace lies with truth. Tell your friend the ANT you are trying to overcome. State the truth you want to believe. Be open about whatever is hard for you. Share the Scripture verse you want to memorize. Try speaking the verse to your friend from memory. Encourage each other in this process. Thank your friend for helping you.

☐ Develop a habit of pausing in the middle of your day and at the end of your day to focus on the replacement thoughts you want to have in your mind in place of your ANTs. Take a minute or two to focus on God's love and care for you. Recite one of the Scripture verses that is helpful to you.

Food Tip
of the Week

To understand what fuels you well and what doesn't, try keeping a food journal. Track what you eat each day to help you identify foods and eating patterns that might be sabotaging your health. Learn more about *The Daniel Plan Journal*, along with an idea for a fruit salad with extra pizzazz. Click the Food Tip of the Week on your video screen (3 minutes), scan the QR code, or go to danielplan.com/foodtip.

Fitness Move
of the Week

You can do this static lunge even if you have back or knee problems. Just click the Fitness Move of the Week on your video screen (1 minute), use the QR code, or go to danielplan.com/fitnessmove.

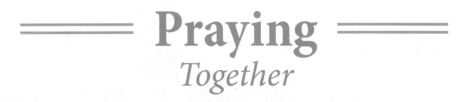

Praying
Together

Because everything we do in our journey toward health depends on God's power, we end each meeting with prayer and encourage group members to pray for each other during the week.

> *"May our Lord Jesus Christ himself and God our Father, who loved us and by his grace gave us eternal encouragement and good hope, encourage your hearts and strengthen you in every good deed and word."*
> 2 Thessalonians 2:16–17

Get into smaller groups of two or three people. Share one ANT you have and the truth you want to believe. Pray for your partner(s) to believe this truth. Pray against anything that would stand in the way of your partner(s) believing that truth.

After you've prayed in smaller groups, have someone close with this prayer:

> *Father, you have promised that the truth will set us free if we question the lies we have believed. Please write the truth on our hearts. Please make us aware each day of the ANTs that infest our minds. Build into us a habitual practice of noticing and questioning our ANTs. Please overcome any resistance inside us to believing the truth. Please guide us to Scripture passages that tell us the truth we need to hear. We know that you are with us, that you will strengthen and help us, that your grace is sufficient for us, and that your power is made perfect in our weakness. Thank you that we can approach your throne of grace with confidence because of Jesus' sacrifice on the cross. I pray this in Jesus' name. Amen.*

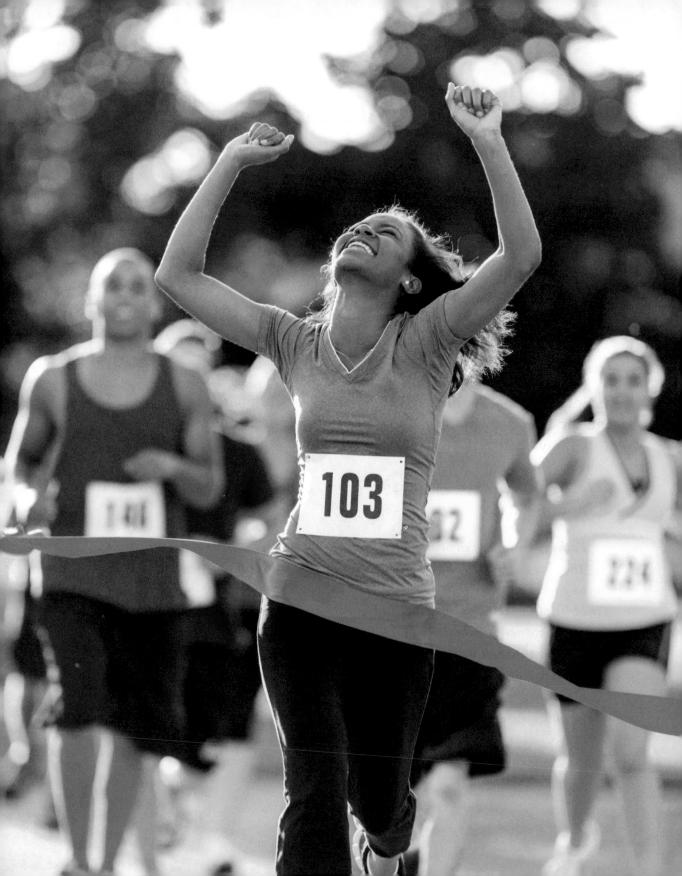

Breaking through Barriers

> "Can anything ever separate us from Christ's love? Does it mean he no longer loves us if we have trouble or calamity, or are persecuted, or hungry, or destitute, or in danger, or threatened with death? . . . No, despite all these things, overwhelming victory is ours through Christ, who loved us."
>
> Romans 8:35, 37 (NLT)

If you've been on The Daniel Plan for more than a couple of weeks, you've probably had some up days and some down days. Everybody has down days, especially early in the process of forming new habits. How can we get something good out of a down day? And how can we interrupt the pattern of persistent down days? Those are the questions we'll address in this session. We'll see how good choices can keep us moving forward through the ups and downs.

COMING
TOGETHER

The other members of your group can be a huge source of support in sustaining healthy changes in your life. Before watching the video, check in with each other about your experiences since the last session. For example:

» Briefly share what Next Steps from Session 2 you completed or tried to complete. Were they helpful? If so, how?

» How did Session 2 affect your thought life?

» Have you been practicing The Daniel Plan in other areas, such as Food or Fitness? If so, what have you done? What is working well for you? What questions do you have? What encouragement do you need?

LEARNING
TOGETHER

AN INTERVIEW WITH Dr. Daniel Amen

Play the video segment for Session 3. As you watch, use the outline provided to follow along or to take additional notes on anything that stands out to you.

»   Everybody fails. Failing is part of learning a new way of life, and The Daniel Plan is a new way of life.

»   Mistakes are simply learning experiences, and there are some things we learn only through failure. We become successful by learning what doesn't work and not doing it anymore. If we're not making any mistakes, we're not growing. So we don't need to be afraid of failure.

»   Turn bad days into good information. Instead of being the victim of your life, be the scientist of your life and study it. If you had a bad day, what happened?

»   One cause of a bad day on The Daniel Plan is second-meal syndrome. Second-meal syndrome says that if we eat badly at breakfast, we are more likely to eat badly at dinner.

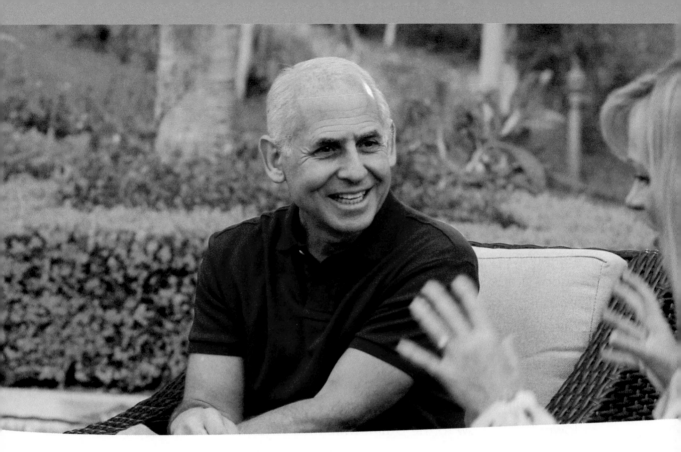

» We also have to be aware of food pushers, people who push us to eat or drink more than or different than we need to eat or drink. Our anxiety can make us worry about "hurting their feelings" if we say no. Instead of saying yes out of anxiety, however, we need to be honest and say something like, "I don't eat like that. My health is critically important to me, and I've learned that if I don't stay on top of it, I can quickly get into a bad habit."

» We need to know what we really want. What are our goals? For example, are weight loss and stable blood sugar truly our goals? Then we need to act in ways that are consistent with our goals.

» Starving ourselves can also lead to failure to live a healthy lifestyle. Diets that seek weight loss by starving ourselves don't work, because when our blood sugar gets too low, we have less blood flow to the part of our brain that helps us make good decisions. We are then more likely to binge on unhealthy foods.

» Eating every three to four hours, and having protein at every meal, keeps blood sugar stable. That leads to better focus and decision making.

» Getting enough sleep is also essential to good decision making. People who get less than six or seven hours of sleep at night have lower blood flow to the brain, which leads to more bad decisions.

» Getting enough vitamin D can also help us avoid failure. When vitamin D levels are low, we become resistant to the hormone leptin, which is supposed to work in the brain to turn off our appetite. When we become leptin resistant, we are hungry all the time. Cravings often go away when we have enough vitamin D. A blood test can determine if we have enough vitamin D.

» ANTs (automatic negative thoughts) can also trigger unhealthy eating, so it's important to address them when they come up.

» Four triggers to poor decisions about food can be remembered with the word HALT:

  • *Hungry.* Don't get too hungry, because if your blood sugar is low, you will make a bad decision.

  • *Angry.* Don't get too angry, because negative thoughts hinder the function of your brain's frontal lobes, so you get confused. Deal with anger constructively. For example, talk to someone who can help you solve the problem. Or have an honest and gracious conversation with the person you are angry at.

  • *Lonely.* Don't get too lonely, because lonely people often eat for comfort. Pursue friendships.

  • *Tired.* Don't go without sleep, because lack of sleep leads to poor decisions.

» A + B = C

  • A is what happens to you. B is how you interpret it. C is how you act. Most people think their actions are determined by what happens to them (they are helpless victims), when in reality how they interpret what happens plays a major role in determining what they do.

  • We need to avoid thinking like victims, blaming someone else for how our lives are turning out. Victims can't change. They are powerless. But in reality, we have the power to decide how to interpret what others do and to decide what we will do in response.

> *"Between stimulus and response there is a space. In that space is our power to choose our response. In our response lies our growth and our freedom."*
> Viktor Frankl, *Man's Search for Meaning*

» When something negative happens, we need to pause, take a deep breath, and reflect. Instead of reacting immediately, we need to think through how we want to respond.

» It's helpful to keep a journal where we can record good days and bad days, to see if we can see patterns of when things began to fall apart. It could be a hormonal issue, or we didn't sleep, or we didn't eat.

» Failure doesn't automatically grow our character. It does so only when we respond to it correctly, when we learn from it, when we say, "What didn't work here, and what can I change?"

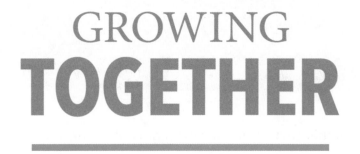

GROWING TOGETHER

Discuss what you learned from the video. Don't feel obliged to answer every question. Select those that most resonate with your group.

1 How is failure an important part of learning a new way of life? What does failure accomplish?

2 How would you go about getting good information from a bad day? What sorts of questions would you ask?

"Rejoice in the Lord always. I will say it again: Rejoice!... Do not be anxious about anything, but in every situation, by prayer and petition, with thanksgiving, present your requests to God. And the peace of God, which transcends all understanding, will guard your hearts and your minds in Christ Jesus."

Philippians 4:4–7

> *"There is no condemnation for those*
> *who belong to Christ Jesus."*
> Romans 8:1 (NLT)

 3 Why is this sort of questioning and reflection more helpful than telling ourselves we deserve condemnation for our failures?

 4 Consider the potential triggers discussed in the Notes section. What do you think might be the top two or three things that can trigger setbacks for you?

☐ Hunger

☐ Anger

☐ Loneliness

☐ Tiredness

☐ Skipping a good breakfast

☐ Not keeping healthy food on hand

☐ Food pushers

☐ ANTs

☐ Stress at work

☐ Lack of nourishment for your soul

☐ Other things (name them):

What can you do about those triggers? (For example, if you tend to get too hungry, you can pack an emergency food pack to keep with you. You can plan ahead to eat healthy food every three to four hours.)

 Explain what A + B = C means. How does it help us avoid thinking like victims?

 How is A + B = C relevant to days when we have setbacks?

"And I am certain that God, who began the good work within you, will continue his work until it is finally finished on the day when Christ Jesus returns."
Philippians 1:6 (NLT)

What I Want
to Remember

Complete this activity on your own.

» Briefly review the video outline and any notes you took. Review also any notes from the discussion.

» In the space below, write down the most significant thing you gained from this session—from the video or the discussion. You can share it with the group if you wish.

BETTER
TOGETHER

Now that you've talked about some great ideas, let's get practical — and put what you're learning into action. Begin by identifying one or two steps you can take in this session on Focus. Then check out the Food Tip of the Week and the Fitness Move of the Week for some fresh ideas to enrich your journey toward health in those areas. Use or adapt whatever is helpful to you!

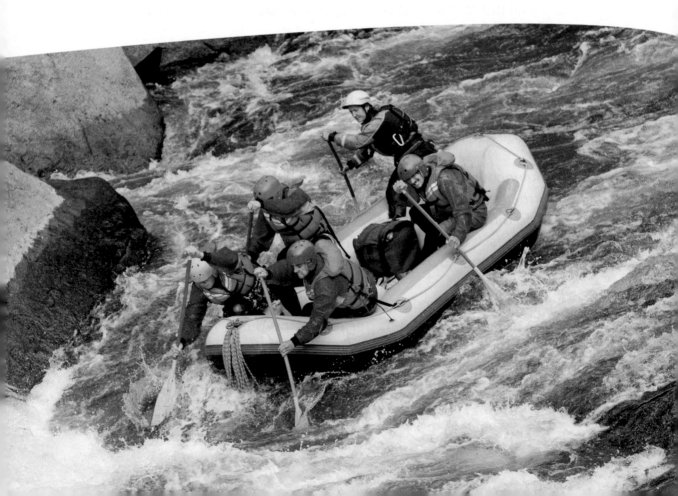

FOCUS
Next Steps

Here are a few suggested activities to help you move forward in dealing with setbacks. Check one or two boxes next to the options you'd like to try this week—choose what works for you.

☐ Practice thinking through your interpretation of an event before you respond to it. When little or big things happen this week, pause and notice yourself interpreting them in a positive or negative light. Ask yourself, "What is the most constructive and helpful way of interpreting this?" Try to put your interpretation into words, especially if you are inclined to respond with anger, fear, shame, or harshness.

☐ If something upsets you this week, write down your interpretation of the event. Then compare your interpretation to the ANTs in the article "Identifying ANTs" in the Appendix. Have you overgeneralized? Are you predicting the future? Are you focusing on the negative? What would be a more constructive way to interpret the event?

☐ If you encounter a setback in your life this week, try examining it for information. What happened? What led to the setback? What could you do differently next time? How can you prepare so that the same thing doesn't happen again? Treat yourself with grace and emphasize information over condemnation.

☐ Start a journal to record good days and bad days on The Daniel Plan. (*The Daniel Plan Journal* is perfect for this purpose.) Write down what you eat for each meal, as well as what you do for exercise each day. You can also include key insights from your devotional time with God and whether you connected with a friend. If you have a bad day, write out what you think led to the setback.

☐ Say no to a food pusher.

☐ Commit yourself to eating a good breakfast each day, with protein and healthy fat rather than sugar or flour.

☐ Commit to getting enough sleep each night this week. How can you shape your routine so that you get to bed at an appropriate hour?

☐ Be aware of times when you are angry this week. Notice how you deal with anger. Do you attack? Do you withdraw? Do you use food to avoid conflict? Do you talk things through rationally? Include in your awareness the milder or more hidden forms of anger, such as irritation, frustration, and boredom.

☐ If loneliness is an issue for you, pursue a friendship. What is something your friend would enjoy doing?

☐ Memorize a verse from this session. See the Memory Verses in the Appendix.

Food Tip
of the Week

Sugar is like poison to our bodies and it dangerously hides in many foods that we innocently eat. This week's food tip is about learning to read labels to uncover the hidden sugar in our diets. Learn what is lurking in your pantry, refrigerator, and freezer. Watch the video, start reading labels, and eliminate the offenders. Just click the Food Tip of the Week on your video screen (3 minutes), scan the QR code, or go to danielplan.com/foodtip.

Fitness Move
of the Week

Try these fun moves *with your eyes closed* to train your balance and give your brain a great workout. Just click the Fitness Move of the Week on your video screen (1 minute), use the QR code, or go to danielplan.com/fitnessmove.

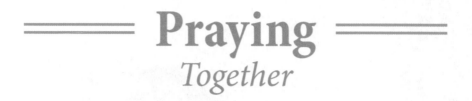

Praying
Together

Because everything we do in our journey toward health depends on God's power, we end each meeting with prayer and encourage group members to pray for each other during the week.

"In repentance and rest is your salvation,
in quietness and trust is your strength."
Isaiah 30:15

Get into smaller groups of two or three people. Share with your partner(s) the things that are most likely to trigger setbacks for you. Is it hunger, anger, loneliness, tiredness, skipping a good breakfast, not keeping healthy food on hand, food pushers, ANTs, stress at work, lack of nourishment for your soul, something else? Then pray for your partner to find effective strategies for dealing with those triggers. Also, pray for your partner(s) to treat themselves gently when they have bad days.

After you've prayed in smaller groups, have someone close with this prayer:

Father, thank you that there is no condemnation for those who belong to Christ Jesus. Thank you that nothing can separate us from your love. We know that you are involved and caring for us in this process of moving toward a healthier lifestyle. Thank you that setbacks aren't evidence of lack of love and involvement on your part. Like King David, we are your servants, born into your household. You have freed us from our chains, and we offer you a sacrifice of thanksgiving. Please give each of us the grace to deal with the things that tend to trigger us to have bad days. Please give us eyes to interpret things that happen to us the way you want us to interpret them. You have graciously honored us with the freedom to choose how we will respond to circumstances, and we ask for the wisdom and strength to interpret and respond well. I pray this in Jesus' name. Amen.

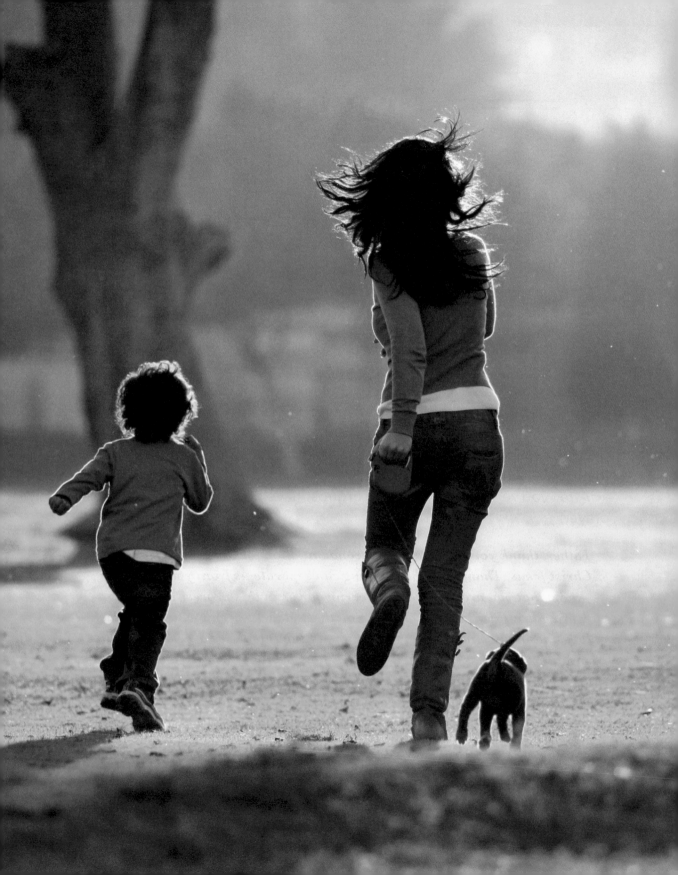

Don't Mess with Stress

> "Give all your worries and cares to God, for he cares about you."
> 1 Peter 5:7 (NLT)

Stress. Everybody faces it. Some of us live under incredible pressure from our circumstances. But we're not in it alone; we have God and each other to support us. Still, we need to establish healthy routines that help us stand up under stress. To replenish ourselves, we need to be intentional as we weave all five of the Essentials into our lifestyle. In this session we'll learn practical strategies to cope and even thrive in a stressful world.

COMING
TOGETHER

The other members of your group can be a huge source of support in sustaining healthy changes in your life. Before watching the video, check in with each other about your experiences since the last session. For example:

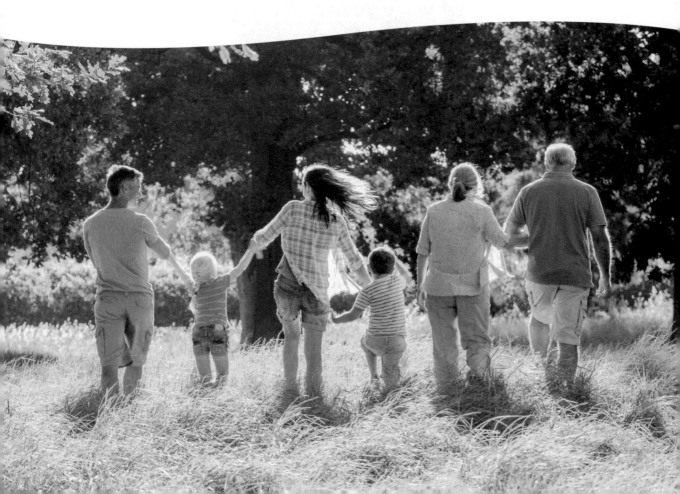

» Briefly share what Next Steps from Session 3 you completed or tried to complete. Were they helpful? If so, how?

» How did Session 3 affect the way you deal with circumstances and setbacks?

» Have you been practicing The Daniel Plan in other areas, such as Food or Fitness? If so, what have you done? What is working well for you? What questions do you have? What encouragement do you need?

LEARNING
TOGETHER

AN INTERVIEW WITH Dr. Daniel Amen

Play the video segment for Session 4. As you watch, use the outline provided to follow along or to take additional notes on anything that stands out to you.

» Many of us face intense stress, and we need to learn how to deal with it, because it has a very negative impact on the body. When the body pumps out stress hormones like cortisol, it decreases the immune system and kills cells in the brain's memory centers.

» If our vitamin D level is good, stress has less of an impact on our bodies. We need an annual blood test for vitamin D.

» We need to know what we want in life, and why. People who have a deep sense of meaning and purpose live 15 percent longer than people who don't. We can write down what we want in our relationships, in work, for our money, for our physical, emotional, and spiritual health. We can write it down and look at it every day.

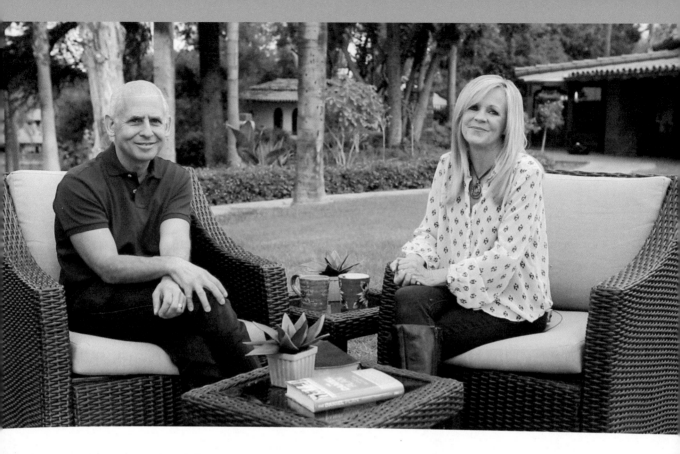

» If we are taking care of the temple that God gave us, then we will have the energy to give back to our families, marriages, ministries, and communities. Intentional living means that we will have the energy to live out our purpose and give back to the world.

» To stop believing the ANTs, we can write them down and question them. "Is it true?" If something upsets us, we can write it down so that we can choose how to interpret it and how we will respond.

» If we graciously weave all five of the Daniel Plan Essentials into our lives, a step at a time, we will have the strong threads that equip us to thrive in difficult seasons.

» A routine of health helps us withstand stress. A little preplanning goes a long way. For example, we need a morning routine of breakfast that emphasizes protein and good fats, not sugar or flour. We also need a routine of exercise. Exercise should be an appointment so that it doesn't get crowded out of our day.

» Don't let grief be an excuse to hurt yourself. There are always excuses for why we hurt ourselves, but don't let them take over. If we make the right choices, we can thrive through the hard times.

» We need to establish a regular weekly Sabbath for worship, rest, and rejoicing. We also need daily Sabbath, times with God throughout the day.

"The LORD is my shepherd, I lack nothing. He makes me lie down in green pastures, he leads me beside quiet waters, he refreshes my soul. He guides me along the right paths for his name's sake. Even though I walk through the darkest valley, I will fear no evil, for you are with me; your rod and your staff, they comfort me. You prepare a table before me in the presence of my enemies. You anoint my head with oil; my cup overflows. Surely your goodness and love will follow me all the days of my life, and I will dwell in the house of the LORD forever."

Psalm 23

"In repentance and rest is your salvation, in quietness and trust is your strength."
Isaiah 30:15

» The secret to happiness is wanting what you have.

» We can overcome so much if we know why we are here and what God wants us to do. But that takes a quiet time during which we actually have communication with God. It can be just a few minutes a day to quiet our minds and ask: Why am I here? What is my purpose? What can I do today in the service of others?

» Time with God can be time spent listening and soaking in God's presence. We don't always have to say a lot of words in prayer. We can soak in the goodness of who God is, enter into his presence, and meditate on a few verses that are replenishing to our souls.

"Be still, and know that I am God."
Psalm 46:10

» So many things in life are out of our control, but the five Essentials are things we can control. We need to be intentional about designing our life with these Essentials and with the dreams and desires we most want to fulfill.

» Breathing from the belly is a good habit for reducing stress. We can breathe in for four slow counts, hold for two, breathe out for four counts, hold for two. Do that for five minutes. Slow breathing like this has been shown to lower people's blood pressure and help their immune systems work better. It helps them make better decisions because it floods their frontal lobes with oxygen so they have more forethought, more judgment, more impulse control.

» We need a rhythm of grace in our lives of slowing down, pausing, entering into God's presence, being still in that place, taking a deep breath, enjoying his goodness, so that we can reboot and move on with our day.

» We also need sleep. If we don't get seven hours of sleep at night, we have lower blood flow to the brain and more bad decisions. Not getting good sleep actually turns off seven hundred health-promoting genes.

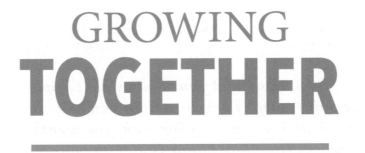

GROWING
TOGETHER

Discuss what you learned from the video. Don't feel obliged to answer every question. Select those that most resonate with your group.

1 On a scale of 1 to 10, with 1 being absolutely no stress and 10 being severe stress, what is the current stress level in your life? What are the causes of your stress, or lack of it?

No stress	1	2	3	4	5	6	7	8	9	10	Severe stress

2 What do you want? Take a moment to write down at least one thing you want in your relationships, your work, your financial goals, or your physical, emotional, or spiritual health. Then share what you wrote with the group if you feel comfortable doing so.

Is it selfish to invest in your physical and mental health? Why or why not? What light does 1 Corinthians 6:19–20 shed on this?

"Do you not know that your bodies are temples of the Holy Spirit, who is in you, whom you have received from God? You are not your own; you were bought at a price. Therefore honor God with your bodies."
1 Corinthians 6:19–20

 What elements can you build into your daily routine to help you withstand stress? Choose two or three elements that you want to prioritize. Look back at the Notes section or ahead to the Next Steps for ideas.

 Why is Sabbath important, both weekly and daily? See Isaiah 30:15 and Psalm 46:10 in the Notes section. (If you want to know more, read the article "Keeping Sabbath" in the Appendix.)

What do you think is the best way for you to practice daily time with God at this stage of your life? What does your soul most need?

What are the most valuable things you have gotten out of this study of Focus? What will you take with you?

What I Want
to Remember

Complete this activity on your own at the end of your group meeting.

» Briefly review the video outline and any notes you took. Review also any notes from the discussion.

» In the space below, write down the most significant thing you gained from this session—from the video or the discussion. You can share it with the group if you wish.

BETTER
TOGETHER

Now that you've talked about some great ideas, let's get practical — and put what you're learning into action. Begin by identifying one or two steps you can take in this session on Focus. Then check out the Food Tip of the Week and the Fitness Move of the Week for some fresh ideas to enrich your journey toward health in those areas. Use or adapt whatever is helpful to you!

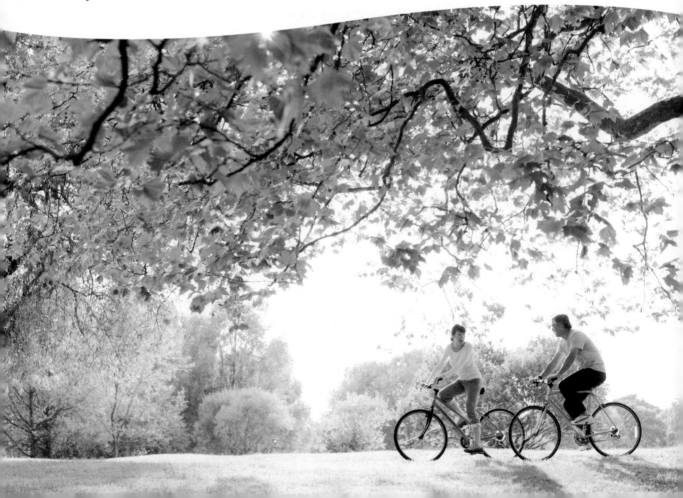

FOCUS
Next Steps

Here are a few suggested activities to help you move forward in dealing with stress. Check one or two boxes next to the options you'd like to try this week—choose what works for you.

- ☐ What do you want? Take some time to write down what you want in your relationships, your work, your financial goals, and your physical, emotional, and spiritual health. Read what you wrote each day this week. If you have trouble putting your goals into words, pair up with a friend to help each other. Explore the question aloud together. Ask your friend for feedback. Write down what you come up with.

- ☐ Commit to a morning routine of breakfast that emphasizes protein and good fats.

- ☐ Make a plan for eating during each weekday. What will you have for lunch? What snacks do you need to have available?

- ☐ Commit to a routine of exercise. Make it an appointment each day.

- ☐ Commit to going to bed at an hour that will give you enough sleep. What adjustments will that require?

- ☐ Continue to question your ANTs.

- ☐ Have daily time with God this week. It can be as simple as taking a break in your day to enter into God's presence, be still in that place, take a deep breath, enjoy his goodness, and meditate on one verse of Scripture. You might read Psalm 23 slowly and pause at a phrase that especially speaks to you. Picture what is described. Stay with the words for a few minutes and let them soak in. You could spend several days with Psalm 23, or go one by one through the Bible passages in this session.

☐ Take a breathing break each day. Breathe in for four slow counts, hold for two counts, breathe out for four counts, hold for two counts. Do this ten times. Try to breathe as deeply and slowly as possible. Fill your belly with breath.

☐ Take a day off from work and chores, a day to worship God and be with family and friends. Take a nap if you need it. Go for a walk. Get outdoors if that replenishes you. Move your body and rest your body. Notice things you're grateful for.

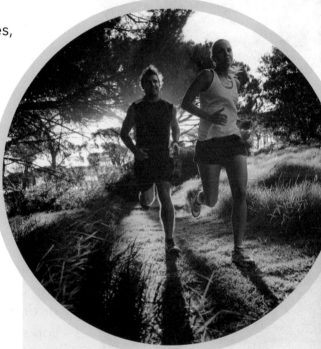

Food Tip
of the Week

Healthy eating does not have to be expensive eating. Learn how to make budget-conscious and health-conscious meals that are wallet friendly. Just click the Food Tip of the Week on your video screen (3 minutes), scan the QR code, or go to danielplan.com/foodtip.

Fitness Move
of the Week

Upper body strength is important for everyday life: carrying children, lifting a vacuum cleaner, or doing yard work. This week's move will help you strengthen your upper body. Just click the Fitness Move of the Week on your video screen (1 minute), use the QR code, or go to danielplan.com/fitnessmove.

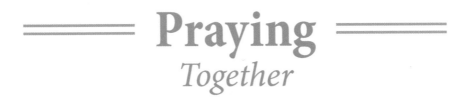

Praying
Together

Because everything we do in our journey toward health depends on God's power, we end each meeting with prayer and encourage group members to pray for each other during the week.

"Be still, and know that I am God."
Psalm 46:10

Give everyone a chance to complete one of these sentences in prayer:

» Lord, one area of stress that I need your help with is _____.

» Lord, one thing I really want (in a relationship, in my work, in my finances, or in my health) is _____.

» Lord, please help me to live intentionally, planning ahead, in the area of _____.

Group members can pray just that one sentence, or they can say more to God on the subject.

Have someone close with this prayer:

Father, we have placed before you the stressors in our lives and the goals we want to pursue. Please fill us with your Holy Spirit so that we will have the strength and patient endurance to thrive in the midst of stress. Please show us what routines you want us to build into our lives so that we can handle stress better. Please hear the things we want and grant them in whatever ways will be best for us. You know what is good for us much better than we do, and you are a generous God who is eager to give. Thank you for all the things we have learned about brain health and governing our thoughts. Please fill our minds with thoughts that honor you. I pray this in Jesus' name. Amen.

Appendix

Biblical Meditation

To meditate is to engage in calm, quiet, and focused thought about something. Biblical meditation does not aim to empty the mind of thoughts. Rather, it aims to focus the mind on thoughts of God. Our minds naturally race along from thought to thought, but when we meditate, we slow down to ponder (carefully weigh), chew on (like a cow chewing its cud), and listen deeply to a small portion of Scripture, a prayer, or a truth about God. We may turn the truth over and over in our minds, to see it from every angle. We may repeat a verse of Scripture to let it sink deeply into our hearts.

Whether or not we are aware of it, we all meditate to some degree. Our minds become stuck on some thought of worry, hurt, anger, or embarrassment. We obsess over it. Or a song gets stuck in our heads. We may want to stop thinking the thought or the song, but we are often powerless to do so unless we have taken the trouble to learn to discipline our thoughts. Practicing deliberate meditation helps us develop the mental muscle to choose what our minds latch onto.

The Bible repeatedly recommends that we learn to meditate on God and his words:

> *"Blessed is the one who does not walk in step with the wicked or stand in the way that sinners take or sit in the company of mockers, but whose delight is in the law of the LORD, and who meditates on his law day and night."*
>
> Psalm 1:1–2

> *"Keep this Book of the Law always on your lips; meditate on it day and night, so that you may be careful to do everything written in it. Then you will be prosperous and successful."*
>
> Joshua 1:8

> *"Within your temple, O God, we meditate on your unfailing love."*
>
> Psalm 48:9

*"I will consider all your works and
meditate on all your mighty deeds."*
Psalm 77:12

"I meditate on your precepts and consider your ways."
Psalm 119:15

*"Cause me to understand the way of your precepts,
that I may meditate on your wonderful deeds."*
Psalm 119:27

*"I reach out for your commands, which I love,
that I may meditate on your decrees."*
Psalm 119:48

*"My eyes stay open through the watches of the night,
that I may meditate on your promises."*
Psalm 119:148

*"Finally, brothers and sisters, whatever is true, what-
ever is noble, whatever is right, whatever is pure, whatever is lovely, whatever is admirable—if anything is
excellent or praiseworthy—think about such things."*
Philippians 4:8

Notice in the above verses that we can meditate on God's words, his love, his deeds, his commands, his promises. We can also meditate on anything that is true and admirable. This doesn't come naturally, but we can learn to do it with practice.

The simplest way to begin is to slowly repeat a verse of Scripture or a true statement over and over in our minds. We may start by reading it aloud until we've memorized it. Then we can repeat it aloud or silently. *Slowly* is important. We want the verse to sink in. We are training our minds to slow down and pay attention.

Here are five other ways to meditate on a verse:

- » **Picture it.** Visualize the scene in your mind.

- » **Pronounce it.** Say the verse aloud, each time emphasizing a different word.

- » **Paraphrase it.** Rewrite the verse in your own words.

- » **Personalize it.** Replace pronouns or people in the verse with your own name.

- » **Pray it.** Turn the verse into a prayer and say it back to God.[*]

The ultimate goal is to get the verse to influence our actions, even when our minds are on other things. Romans 12:1 speaks of this as being transformed by the renewing of our minds. Our minds are renewed, and our actions follow.

Many of the Fitness Moves of the Week in this series invite us to stand in a posture or do a movement while meditating on a Scripture verse. We will inevitably think about something while we do the move for a full minute, so it might as well be something that strengthens our souls while the move strengthens our bodies.

What should we meditate on? Two passages we might start with are Psalm 23 and Romans 8:31 – 39. Take them a verse at a time. If you want something shorter, try one of these:

"Truly my soul finds rest in God; my salvation comes from him. Truly he is my rock and my salvation; he is my fortress, I will never be shaken."

Psalm 62:1 – 2

"So do not fear, for I am with you; do not be dismayed, for I am your God. I will strengthen you and help you; I will uphold you with my righteous right hand."

Isaiah 41:10

---

[*] Rick Warren, *Rick Warren's Bible Study Methods: Twelve Ways You Can Unlock God's Word* (Grand Rapids: Zondervan, 2012), 41 – 43.

"But [God] said to me, 'My grace is sufficient for you, for my power is made perfect in weakness.' Therefore I will boast all the more gladly about my weaknesses, so that Christ's power may rest on me."
2 Corinthians 12:9

"Come to me, all you who are weary and burdened, and I will give you rest. Take my yoke upon you and learn from me, for I am gentle and humble in heart, and you will find rest for your souls. For my yoke is easy and my burden is light."
Matthew 11:28–30

"The LORD your God is with you, the Mighty Warrior who saves. He will take great delight in you; in his love he will no longer rebuke you, but will rejoice over you with singing."
Zephaniah 3:17

"Let us then approach God's throne of grace with confidence, so that we may receive mercy and find grace to help us in our time of need."
Hebrews 4:16

"Take delight in the LORD, and he will give you the desires of your heart."
Psalm 37:4

Other things to meditate on include:

» The good things God has done for you and your loved ones

» Jesus' willingness to become human for your sake (John 1:14)

» Jesus' willingness to suffer for your sake

» Anything God has recently taught you

There's an old saying, "You are what you eat." That's true of our minds as well as our bodies: we are what we feed our minds. Be sure to feed your mind a healthy diet of Scripture.

Identifying ANTs

Therapists have identified several kinds of negative thoughts that keep people stuck in bad habits. Use these categories to identify your ANTs.

1. Overgeneralization. This usually involves thoughts with words like *always, never, every time*, or *everyone* and makes a situation out to be worse than it really is. Here are some examples:

> » *I have always been fat; it will never change.*

> » *Every time I get stressed, I have to eat something.*

> » *I don't like any of the foods that are good for me.*

Overgeneralizations make you believe you have no control over your actions and that you are incapable of changing your behaviors.

2. Thinking with your feelings. These negative thoughts occur when you have a feeling about something and you assume your feeling is correct. Feelings are complex and are often rooted in powerful memories from the past. Feelings, like thoughts, can lie. These thoughts usually begin with the words "I feel." For example:

> » *I feel like a failure.*

> » *I feel God has abandoned me.*

> » *I feel hungry and must eat or I will get sick.*

Whenever you have a strong negative feeling, check it out. Look for the evidence behind the feeling. Is it based on events or experiences from the past?

3. Predicting the future. Predicting the worst in a situation causes an immediate sense of anxiety, which can trigger cravings for sugar or refined carbs and make you feel that you need to eat to calm your nerves. What makes future-telling so toxic is that your mind tends to make happen what it sees.

> » *Healthy food will be expensive, taste like cardboard, and won't fill me up.*

> » *I can't change my habits for the long term.*

> » *My spouse or kids will never do this with me.*

4. Blame. When you blame something or someone else for the problems in your life, you become a victim of circumstances, as though you can't do anything to change your situation. Be honest and ask yourself if you have a tendency to say things such as . . .

> » *It's your fault I'm out of shape because you won't exercise with me.*

> » *It's not my fault I eat too much; my mom taught me to clean my plate.*

> » *If restaurants didn't give such big servings, I wouldn't be so overweight.*

> » *I'm overweight because of my genetics.*

5. Focusing on the negative. Some people can take any positive experience and taint it with something negative. For instance:

> » *I wanted to lose thirty pounds in ten weeks, but I have only lost eight pounds. I'm a complete failure.*

> » *I went to the gym and did a hard workout, but the guy on the bike next to me was talking the whole time, so I'm never going back there.*

> » *I started eating two servings of vegetables a day, but I should be eating five for optimal health, so why bother?*

Keeping Sabbath

When God created the world, he worked for six days and then took a day to rest and enjoy what he had made (Genesis 2:1–3). When he freed his chosen people from slavery in Egypt, he commanded them to keep the seventh day holy, set apart as a day of rest (Exodus 20:8–11). That day of rest, that Sabbath, had several purposes. It was a way of honoring God as Creator. It respected the people's human limitations as creatures made in God's image to work and rest. And it celebrated their liberation from slavery (Deuteronomy 5:15). Slaves never get a day off, but free people do.

The Jewish Sabbath is on the seventh day, Saturday. It is a day for worship, rest, and rejoicing. But soon after Jesus' resurrection from the dead, the early Christians adopted the day of his rising, Sunday, as their day for worship and rejoicing. Few Christians living under Roman rule were able to take either Saturday or Sunday as a day of rest, because their masters and their society expected them to work every day. Not until AD 321 did the Roman emperor Constantine make Sunday a day of rest in the empire.

God saw the Sabbath as so important that he included it as one of the Ten Commandments. Yet today, Christians who would never break the commandments about adultery or murder often treat the commandment about Sabbath as a luxury of a bygone era. Many Christians work long hours during the week and take Sunday as a day for shopping and household chores. And if Sunday is a shopping day, retail workers have to work on Sundays. Office workers, too, find that their supervisors email them on weekends or expect more to get done than six days can hold. Our society no longer has a day of rest, and it's hard for individuals and families to swim against that tide.

Yet we need Sabbaths for worship, rest, and rejoicing. We need to be reminded that God is the one who makes food crops grow and provides jobs and paychecks. We need a day away from labor and buying and selling, a day to cultivate nonmaterial things. We need a day with our loved ones, a long walk or bike ride, or a few hours alone. We need to stop living as slaves.

How can you make a weekly Sabbath part of your family's practice? How can you say no to work and shopping one day a week, in order to worship, exercise, get out in nature, take a nap, enjoy a meal with family and friends, or get alone with God?

In addition to a weekly Sabbath, we also need daily time to be refreshed by our relationship with God. He says, "Be still, and know that I am God" (Psalm 46:10). It's a good idea to set aside some time each morning, or at midday, or in the evening for that stillness with God. We might reflect on a small portion of Scripture, offer our prayer requests, and ask God to show us how to do his will today.

Psalm 23:3 says that God restores and refreshes our souls. He longs to do that for us, and keeping Sabbath — both daily and weekly — is one of the best things we can do to let him give us that refreshment.

Group Guidelines

Our goal: To provide a safe environment where participants experience authentic community and spiritual growth.

OUR VALUES	
Group Attendance	To give priority to the group meeting. We will call or email if we will be late or absent.
Safe Environment	To help create a safe place where people can be heard and feel loved.
Respect Differences	To be gentle and gracious to people with different spiritual maturity, personal opinions, or personalities. Remember we are all works in progress!
Confidentiality	To keep anything that is shared strictly confidential and within the group, and to avoid sharing information about those outside the group.
Encouragement for Growth	We want to spiritually multiply our life by serving others with our God-given gifts.
Rotating Hosts/Leaders and Homes	To encourage different people to host the group in their homes, and to rotate the responsibility of facilitating each meeting.

We have found that groups thrive when they talk about expectations up front and come into agreement on some of these details listed below.

Refreshments/mealtimes _____

Child care _____

When we will meet (day of week) _____

Where we will meet (place) _____

We will begin at (time) _____ and end at _____

We will look for a compatible time to attend a worship service together.

Our primary worship service time will be _____

Leadership 101

Congratulations! You have responded to the call to help shepherd Jesus' flock. There are few other tasks in the family of God that surpass the contribution you will be making. As you prepare to lead, whether it is one session or four, here are a few thoughts to keep in mind. We encourage you to read these and review them with each new discussion leader before he or she leads.

1. **Remember that you are not alone.** God knows everything about you, and he knew that you would be asked to lead your group. It is common for leaders to feel that they are not ready to lead. Moses, Solomon, Jeremiah, Timothy—they all were reluctant to lead. God promises, "Never will I leave you; never will I forsake you" (Hebrews 13:5). You will be blessed as you serve.

2. **Don't try to do it alone.** Pray right now for God to help you build a healthy leadership team. If you can enlist a co-leader to help you lead the group, you will find your experience to be much richer. That person might take half the group in a second discussion circle if your group is as large as ten people or more. Your co-leader might lead the prayer time or handle the hosting tasks, welcoming people and getting them refreshments. This is your chance to involve as many people as you can in building a healthy group. All you have to do is call and ask people to help; you'll be surprised at the response.

3. **Just be yourself.** God wants you to use your unique gifts and temperament. Don't try to do things exactly like another leader; do them in a way that fits you! Just admit it when you don't have an answer, and apologize when you make a mistake. Your group will love you for it, and you'll sleep better at night.

4. **Prepare for your meeting ahead of time.** Review the session, view the video, and write down your responses to each question. If paper and pens are needed, such as for gathering group members' names and email addresses (see "Coming Together" in Session 1), be sure you have the necessary supplies. Think about which "Next Steps" you will do.

   If you're leading Session 1, look over the Group Guidelines and be ready to review them with the group. If child care will be an issue for your group, for example, be prepared to talk about options. Some groups have the adults share the cost of a babysitter (or two) to care for children in a different part of the house where the adults are meeting. Other groups use one home for the kids and another for the adults. A third idea is to rotate the responsibility of caring for the children in the same home or one nearby.

5. **Pray for your group members by name.** Before you begin your session, go around the room in your mind and pray for each member. You may want to review the group's prayer list at least once a week. Ask God to use your time together to work in the heart of each person uniquely. Expect God to lead you to whomever he wants you to encourage or challenge in a special way.

6. **When you ask a question, be patient.** Read each question aloud and wait for someone to respond. Sometimes people need a moment or two of silence to think about the question, and if silence doesn't bother you, it won't bother anyone else. After someone responds, affirm the response with a simple "thanks" or "good job." Then ask, "How about somebody else?" or "Would someone who hasn't shared like to add anything?" Be sensitive to new people or reluctant members who aren't ready to participate yet. If you give them a safe setting, they will open up over time. Don't go around the circle and have everyone answer every question. Your goal is a conversation in which the group members talk to each other in a natural way.

7. **Break up into small groups each week or people won't stay.** If your group has more than eight people, we strongly encourage you to have the group gather sometimes in discussion circles of three or four people during the "Growing Together" section of the study. With a greater opportunity to talk in a small circle, people will connect more with the study, apply more quickly what they are learning, and ultimately get more out of it. A small circle also encourages a quiet person to participate and tends to minimize the effect of a more vocal or dominant member. It can also help people feel more loved in your group. When you gather again at the end of the section, you can have one person summarize the highlights from each circle.

    Small circles are also helpful during prayer time. People who are not accustomed to praying aloud will feel more comfortable trying it with just two or three others. Also, prayer requests won't take as much time, so circles will have more time to actually pray. When you gather back with the whole group, you can have one person from each circle briefly update everyone on the prayer requests.

8. **One final challenge for new leaders:** Before your opportunity to lead, look up each of the four passages listed below. Read each one as a devotional exercise to help equip you with a shepherd's heart. If you do this, you will be more than ready for your first meeting.

    Matthew 9:36
    1 Peter 5:2-4
    Psalm 23
    Ezekiel 34:11-16

For additional tips and resources, go to danielplan.com/tools.

Memory Verses

SESSION 1

"Rejoice always, pray continually, give thanks in all circumstances; for this is God's will for you in Christ Jesus."

1 Thessalonians 5:16-18

SESSION 2

"Finally, brothers and sisters, whatever is true, whatever is noble, whatever is right, whatever is pure, whatever is lovely, whatever is admirable—if anything is excellent or praiseworthy—think about such things."

Philippians 4:8

SESSION 3

"And I am certain that God, who began the good work within you, will continue his work until it is finally finished on the day when Christ Jesus returns."

Philippians 1:6 (NLT)

SESSION 4

"You will keep in perfect peace all who trust in you, all whose thoughts are fixed on you!"

Isaiah 26:3 (NLT)

About the Contributors

GUEST SPEAKERS

Daniel Amen, MD is a physician, a double board certified psychiatrist and a Distinguished Fellow of the American Psychiatric Association, neuroscientist, and nine-time *New York Times* bestselling author. He is the Founder and Medical Director of Amen Clinics in Newport Beach and San Francisco, California; Bellevue, Washington; Reston, Virginia; Atlanta; and New York City. Dr. Amen's extensive research and innovative approach to optimizing the brain has helped millions of people worldwide.

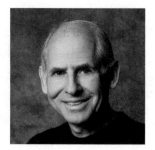

Dee Eastman is the Founding Director of The Daniel Plan that has helped over 15,000 people lose 260,000 pounds in the first year alone. Dee completed her education in Health Science with an emphasis in long-term lifestyle change. Her experience in corporate wellness and ministry has fueled her passion to help people transform their health while drawing closer to God. She coauthored the *Doing Life Together* Bible study series and was a contributing author of *The Daniel Plan*.

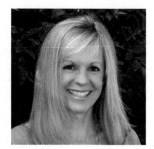

SIGNATURE CHEFS

Sally Cameron is a professional chef, author, recipe developer, educator, certified health coach, and one of the contributors to *The Daniel Plan Cookbook*. Sally's passion is to inspire people to create great-tasting meals at home using healthy ingredients and easy techniques. Sally is the publisher of the popular food blog, *A Food Centric Life*. She holds a culinary degree from The Art Institute and health coaching certification from The Institute for Integrative Nutrition.

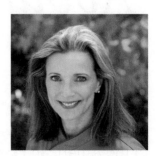

Jenny Ross is the internationally recognized chef, author, educator, and force behind Jenny Ross Living Foods, including the raw food restaurant 118 Degrees, the popular Raw Basics detox meal programs, and nationwide grocery product line 118 Degrees. She has been an early pioneer of the raw movement, coaching clients about the healing power of living foods, while motivating them to adopt a more vibrant, healthy lifestyle. She has a degree in holistic nutrition and certificates as a health and life coach. Jenny was one of the contributing chefs of *The Daniel Plan Cookbook*.

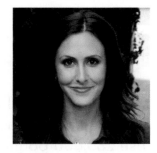

FITNESS TEAM

Sean Foy is an internationally renowned authority on fitness, weight management, and healthy living. As an author, exercise physiologist, behavioral coach, and speaker, Sean has earned the reputation as "America's Fast Fitness Expert." With an upbeat and sensible approach to making fitness happen, he's taken the message of "simple moves" fitness all over the world. Sean is the author of *Fitness That Works, Walking 4 Wellness, The Burst Workout,* and a contributing author *The Daniel Plan.*

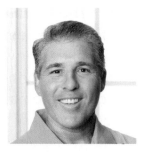

Basheerah Ahmad is a well-known celebrity fitness expert, with a heart for serving God's people. Whether it be through television appearances (*Dr. Phil, The Doctors*), writing fitness and nutrition books, speaking publicly about health, or teaching classes in under-served communities, Basheerah has dedicated her life to improving the health of people everywhere. She has a MS in Exercise Science and numerous certifications in fitness and nutrition. She was a lead fitness instructor for *The Daniel Plan in Action* fitness video series.

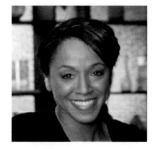

Tony "The Marine" Lattimore is one of Southern California's premier fitness experts. A skilled personal trainer who privately trains professional athletes, celebrities, and community leaders, he has competed nationally as a bodybuilder. Tony's fitness expertise was featured in P90X and *The Daniel Plan in Action* fitness video series. His powerhouse workouts have a reputation for making fitness fun and exhilarating.

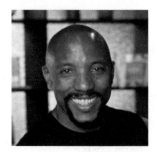

Kevin Forbes has a passion for inspiring others to build healthy habits and push through their physical and mental boundaries. Kevin has helped others grow as a personal trainer, group fitness instructor, and fitness professional. Most recently, he was a featured fitness instructor in *The Daniel Plan in Action* fitness video series. Kevin mentors not only future fitness leaders but also the foster youth in his local community.

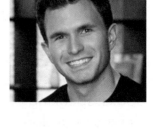

Janet Hertogh shares her love and enthusiasm for teaching in the classroom as an elementary school teacher and in a variety of fitness classes at Saddleback Church. Her passion for life change and transformation is a central theme wherever she goes. Her Masters Degree in Education along with her AFAA and personal training certification make her fully equipped to influence many. Janet was a featured fitness instructor in *The Daniel Plan in Action* fitness video series.

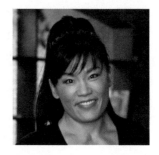

The Daniel Plan

40 Days to a Healthier Life

Rick Warren D. Min., Daniel Amen M.D., Mark Hyman M.D.

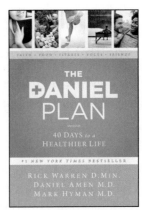

Revolutionize Your Health ... Once and for All.

During an afternoon of baptizing over 800 people, Pastor Rick Warren realized it was time for change. He told his congregation he needed to lose weight and asked if anyone wanted to join him. He thought maybe 200 people would sign up; instead he witnessed a movement unfold as 15,000 people lost over 260,000 pounds in the first year. With assistance from medical and fitness experts, Pastor Rick and thousands of people began a journey to transform their lives.

Welcome to The Daniel Plan.

Here's the secret sauce: The Daniel Plan is designed to be done in a supportive community relying on God's instruction for living.

When it comes to getting healthy, two are always better than one. Our research has revealed that people getting healthy together lose twice as much weight as those who do it alone. God never meant for you to go through life alone and that includes the journey to health.

Unlike the thousands of other books on the market, this book is not about a new diet, guilt-driven gym sessions, or shame-driven fasts. *The Daniel Plan* shows you how the powerful combination of faith, fitness, food, focus, and friends will change your health forever, transforming you in the most head-turning way imaginably—from the inside out.

Available in stores and online!

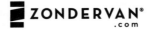

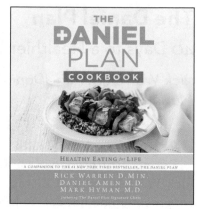

THE ✚DANIEL PLAN

The Daniel Plan Cookbook

Healthy Eating for Life

Rick Warren D. Min., Daniel Amen M.D., and Mark Hyman M.D. featuring The Daniel Plan Signature Chefs

Based on *The Daniel Plan* book, *The Daniel Plan Cookbook: 40 Days to a Healthier Life* is a beautiful four-color cookbook filled with more than 100 delicious, Daniel Plan-approved recipes that offer an abundance of options to bring healthy cooking into your kitchen.

No boring drinks or bland entrées here. Get ready to enjoy appetizing, inviting, clean, simple meals to share in community with your friends and family.

Healthy cooking can be easy and delicious, and *The Daniel Plan Cookbook* is the mouth-watering companion to *The Daniel Plan* book and *The Daniel Plan Journal* to help transform your health in the most head-turning way imaginably—from the inside out.

Available in stores and online!

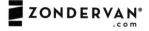

THE DANIELPLAN

The Daniel Plan Journal

40 Days to a Healthier Life

Rick Warren and The Daniel Plan Team

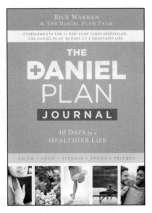

The Perfect Daniel Plan Companion for Better Overall Health

Research shows that tracking your food and exercise greatly contributes to your long-term success. Maximize your momentum by exploring and charting your journey through the five key Essentials of The Daniel Plan—Faith, Food, Fitness, Focus, and Friends.

Taking readers of *The Daniel Plan: 40 Days to a Healthier Life* to the next level, *The Daniel Plan Journal* is the perfect companion, providing encouraging reminders about your health. On the days you need a little boost, *The Daniel Plan Journal* has the daily Scripture, inspiration, and motivation you need to stay on track and keep moving forward.

Available in stores and online!

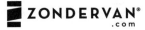

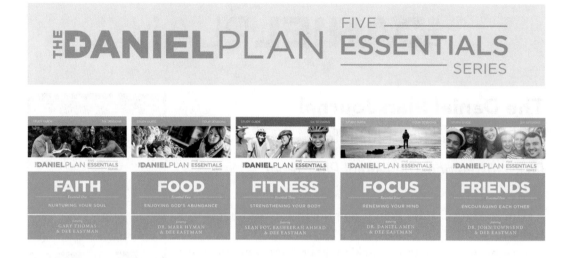

The Daniel Plan Five Essentials Series

The Daniel Plan Five Essentials Series is an innovative approach to creating a healthy lifestyle, rooted and framed by five life areas: Faith, Food, Fitness, Focus, and Friends.

Host Dee Eastman and The Daniel Plan's founding doctors and wellness faculty — including Gary Thomas, Dr. Mark Hyman, Sean Foy, Basheerah Ahmad, Dr. Daniel Amen, and Dr. John Townsend — equip you to make healthy choices on a daily basis.

Each video session features not only great teaching but testimony from those who have incorporated The Daniel Plan into their everyday lives. A weekly Fitness Move and Food Tip are also provided. The study guide include icebreakers and review questions, video notes, video discussion questions, next steps suggestions, prayer starters, and helpful appendices.

The Daniel Plan has transformed thousands of people around the world and it can transform you as well.

Available in stores and online!

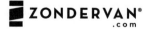

The Daniel Plan in Action

40 Day Fitness Programs With Dynamic Workouts

Introduction by Rick Warren D. Min.

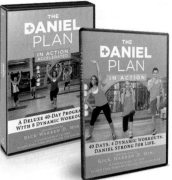

The Daniel Plan in Action is a 40-day fitness system with an innovative approach to creating a healthy lifestyle, rooted and framed by five life areas: faith, food, fitness, focus and friends. Three expert instructors lead the variety of inspiring workouts with a strong backbone of faith and community, complemented by a soundtrack of exclusive Christian music. This 4-session and 8-session systems focus on an abundance of healthy choices offering you the encouragement and inspiration you need to succeed.

Go to DanielPlan.com now to learn more.

The Daniel Plan Jumpstart Guide

Daily Steps to a Healthier Life

*Rick Warren D. Min., Daniel Amen M.D.,
Mark Hyman M.D.*

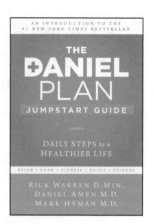

The Daniel Plan Jumpstart Guide provides a bird's-eye view of getting your life on track to better health in five key areas: Faith, Food, Fitness, Focus, and Friends. This booklet provides all the key principles for readers to gain a vision for health and get started — breaking out existing content from *The Daniel Plan: 40 Days to a Healthier Life* into a 40-day action plan. The *Jumpstart Guide* encourages readers to use *The Daniel Plan* and *The Daniel Plan Journal* for more information and further success.

Available in stores and online!

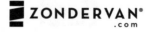